Fueling Male Fertility

Nutrition and Lifestyle Guidance for Men Trying to Conceive

Lauren Manaker MS, RDN, LD, CLEC

Note: This guide is not intended as a substitute for medical advice from a physician. It offers information and guidance based on scientific studies and professional experience. No outcome is promised. Ideally, a focus on overall good health may benefit any read

CONTENTS

CONTENTS

ACKNOWLEDGMENTS

My hope is that this guide will being couples one step closer to expanding their families.
I am grateful to have had such support during the creation of this guide.

My grandfather Paul Niloff MD graciously offered his insight and expertise when the goals of this guide were being established.

Bootsie Terry not only offered her proofreading expertise, but was a fabulous cheerleader during this process.

Melissa Groves RDN was so kind to review the content of this guide and offered her professional opinion which was invaluable.

I cannot imagine a better editor to work with, and am so glad that I had an opportunity to work with Linda Ingroia. Working with her made this process run smoothly and (dare I say) fun!

My sister Samantha was my cheerleader throughout this process. She gave me her time, insight, and encouragement and I am so thankful.

Annie Grotophorst is the most gifted graphic designer and I am so excited that she was willing to create the cover for this guide. Thank you for your creativity and expertise.

1 INTRODUCTION

The groundwork of all happiness is health. ~ **James Leigh Hunt**

Although conventional wisdom might seem to be that infertility is a female problem, in fact, it's not a woman's alone; an increasing collection of research confirms the saying that "it takes two to tango" when it comes to fertility. After all, half of the baby's origins and genetic makeup will be coming from the man.

In 2018, the Center for Disease Control and Prevention issued a report stating that total fertility rates in the United States (estimated number of lifetime births expected per 1,000 women) fell 18 percent in large metro counties and 16 percent in small or medium metro counties between 2007 and 2017.[1] One in eight couples in the United States has trouble getting pregnant or sustaining a pregnancy.[2] Globally, infertility affects an estimated 15% of couples.[3]

In fact, these problems are equally distributed between males and females.[4] Overall, one third of infertility cases are caused by male reproductive issues, one third by female reproductive issues, and one third by both male and female reproductive issues or by unknown factors.[5]

Whether you and your partner are having trouble conceiving or are just considering starting a family, a man's contribution and therefore a man's health is an important influence to consider.

A man's diet and lifestyle choices can affect his health, including his sperm and hormone production. When a couple struggles with infertility, the man modifying certain lifestyle practices is one thing that he can do that may help the conception process.

Increasing evidence suggests that certain dietary and lifestyle practices may enhance male fertility, while other practices may hinder it.

PURPOSE OF THIS GUIDE

My goal with this guide is to provide men (or women with male partners or a known sperm donor) with the most up-to-date, evidence-based, and practical information available so you can be informed and, if necessary, take action to improve your health.

In my role as a nutrition counselor, I have female clients who ask for advice regarding improving or maintaining fertility but I rarely have male clients with the same request. Although this evidence is anecdotal, I also find that women say their husbands don't like to visit doctors or health professionals in general, and feel that diet and lifestyle issues are health "light" and they can investigate these issues on their own.

However, the internet is both a blessing and a curse. Information is easily accessible, but often it comes from unreliable sources. Additionally, well-meaning friends or family members offer advice that may not be the most accurate or relevant to your situation.

There are currently no easy, clear clinical guidelines for male patients seeking fertility treatment.[6] However, in this book, I help you separate the real information from the ridiculous.

Specifically, this guide will:

1. Provide an understanding of the man's role in reproduction, and how his lifestyle plays a role in couples becoming pregnant.
2. Offer the evidence that supports potential enhancement of male fertility through diet and lifestyle, which may be the missing link of why couples are unsuccessful at conceiving.
3. Showcase in a simple format the proven, basic changes you can make to your diet and lifestyle to help you achieve your goals based on any specific diagnosis you may have (like low sperm count, etc.). No gimmicks, just science.

To provide the most applicable information, I try to focus on recent data and only provide information based on research concerning humans (no rats, monkeys, or chickens!).

WHAT YOU CAN CONTROL

Fertility is influenced by many things and nutrition and lifestyle are small components in the big picture. There may be a chromosomal or physical abnormality, medication mismanagement, or other factors that are out of your personal control. However, nutrition and lifestyle choices ARE in your control. Making any of these dietary or lifestyle changes should not *decrease* your chances of becoming pregnant as a couple. You have to eat anyway, so why not eat and live in a way that has been shown to support your goals?

A note about diet supplements and herbal remedies: In my work as a registered dietitian and in this book, I don't focus much on supplement recommendations or herbs. Given the fact that some companies sell fertility "miracle pills," I was shocked to find very few human studies that support their claims. While some of these remedies have been featured in animal studies and they serve their purpose in the research world, I reserve my recommendations to those supported by human studies. Human anatomy and physiology differ from that for animals that have been studied.

Essentially, this is a guide with straightforward, simple approaches and tweaks that can be incorporated into most people's diets and lifestyles at your own pace and with your own control. Of course, any personalized information you receive from your doctor, dietitian, or other health care provider should be followed first.

This guide is not a substitute for any accredited health provider's care.

EATING FOR TWO

"Eating for two" is something you and your partner can both do to set the stage for a healthy pregnancy. It can ideally lead to a quick and successful conception stage. It is something that can be also be done to show support for your female partner and establish that you both are committed to a successful outcome.

After all, experts have stated that: "The nutritional status of both women and men before conception has profound implications for the growth, development, and long-term health of their offspring."[7] Planning pregnancy is very important to ensure the most comfortable and optimal conditions for conception, gestation, and the subsequent birth of a healthy child.[8]

Generally speaking, it is recommended to begin healthy practices three months before you hope to conceive, what is known as the "preconception period".[9] For men, you want to avoid taking anything that may negatively affect spermatogenesis (sperm production). The entire process of spermatogenesis takes on average 64 days.[10]

Therefore, if a man is planning on "eating for two," he should plan on doing this at least 64 days before, or a little over two months before trying to conceive.

What You will Find In This Guide

In this guide, you will find specific nutrition and lifestyle interventions that have been shown to improve male fertility parameters in scientific peer-reviewed papers. You will also find my personal recommendations for how to implement certain measures. Lastly, you will find a brief outline highlighting certain things you can do to modify your diet and lifestyle according to specific fertility challenges.

2 WHY SHOULD MEN CARE ABOUT FERTILITY?

You Matter.

Beyond the fun involved in "making babies," men have considerable influence beyond the "act" on actually making conception a reality and developing a healthy child.

Scientific research shows that your nutrition status at the time of conception can impact all of those outcomes!

It's true, though, that many people only take interest once there is a problem. So, here's the latest about the problem: In 2018, the fertility rate in the United States fell to 60.2 births per 1,000 women of childbearing age, down 3 percent from 2016. In 2017, couples had nearly 500,000 fewer babies than in 2007, despite the fact that there were an estimated 7 percent more women in their prime childbearing years of 20 to 39.[2] As mentioned previously, one in eight couples struggle with infertility.[2]

This may partly speak to people making a choice not to have children, but it largely reflects infertility issues. And according to several studies, approximately 40-50% of infertility cases are due to a male factor.[3,11]

Male infertility may be from one or a combination of low sperm concentration, poor sperm motility, abnormal morphology, or other issues.[11]

For example, between 1973 and 2011, research has shown an approximate 50 percent decrease in sperm counts in Western countries based on an analysis of 185 studies.[12]

To evaluate male fertility, a medical history and physical examination and at least two semen analyses (SAs) should be obtained.[13] The semen analyses should be conducted at least seven days apart and within two or three months.

A semen analysis will assess many factors that may affect male fertility. Here's the low-down on issues that could come up.

SPERM CONCERNS

Low Sperm Count (Oligospermia).

Low sperm count means there is a lower amount of sperm per sample than what is established as ideal.

The World Health Organization (WHO) classifies ideal sperm counts at or above 15 million sperm per milliliter (mL) of semen as an average.[14] A low sperm count does not necessarily mean the man will not be able to get his partner pregnant. It simply may mean that it takes more "tries" and time before success is seen.

Poor Movement/Motility (Asthenozoospermia)

Poor sperm motility means that the sperm do not swim properly.

Asthenozoospermia is diagnosed when less than 32 percent of the sperm is able to move efficiently, and this must be measured within 60 minutes of collection.[14] If sperm do not swim properly, they may have trouble getting to the egg and therefore assisted reproduction technology may need to be explored.

Low Semen Volume (hypospermia)

Low semen volume refers to when a an produces a lower-than-normal volume of semen, or ejaculate. WHO regards 1.5 ml as the lower reference limit.[14]

Hypospermia should not be confused with oligospermia, or low sperm count. Hypospermia would only usually be considered a factor in infertility if both tests for both conditions (hypospermia and oligospermia) reflected concerning numbers.[15]

Abnormal Sperm Shape/Morphology (Teratozoospermia)

Abnormal sperm shape means that a statistically significant percentage of sperm has abnormal size and shape. The sperm may demonstrate features such as more than one head, misshaped head, or more than one tail.

Abnormal sperm morphology might affect the ability of the sperm to reach and penetrate an egg.

Certain conditions may not be as much of concern in certain situations. For example, if a man has a low sperm motility but a high sperm count, the motility may not play as much of a negative role in potential fertility struggles.

Sperm DNA Fragmentation or Damage

DNA is the carrier of genetic information, so having sperm with intact DNA is key. Sperm DNA contributes half of the offspring's genetic material. If the DNA is damaged, abnormal, or fragmented (broken), it may affect pregnancy success.

The DNA in sperm is protected inside the sperm

head. If it is protected well, some theorize that the DNA is protected from molecules called free radicals that may damage the DNA[16] (more on that later!).

HORMONAL ISSUES/TESTOSTERONE

Testosterone is a key male hormone. Among its many roles, it plays a part in sperm production. If a man has a low testosterone level, he may have fertility challenges due to altered sperm production or lower libido (which may result in challenges to "trying").

Men may think that a testosterone replacement therapy is essential if they are dealing with low testosterone levels. However, this intervention has been shown to reduce sperm count in men due to its effect on other hormones[17], and it is not recommended to utilize this therapy without consulting your health care provider.

There are other methods for rebalancing testosterone levels that have been shown to be an effective choice for men trying to conceive and should be discussed with your health care provider.

It is not advised to use testosterone replacement therapy without your doctor's consent, especially if you are trying to conceive.

3 DIET AND LIFESTYLE FACTORS THAT AFFECT MALE FERTILITY

"A man too busy to take care of his health is like a mechanic too busy to take care of his tools." ~Spanish proverb

There are four factors that have been hypothesized to play a role in male fertility. If one element is off balance, it could affect the big picture. The four most influential lifestyle factors on health are:

- Diet
- Tobacco and drugs
- Exercise
- Stress[18]

When trying to conceive, men should try to manage these four elements, especially if he has been diagnosed with male-factor infertility. Although this guide is heavily focused on diet, the other three factors will be discussed as well.

4 OBESITY

Obesity rates in the United States are on the rise.
Almost 40% of the US population was considered
obese in a 2015-2016 survey according to the Center
for Disease Control and Prevention.[19] If your body
mass index, or BMI, is 30 or higher, you are
considered obese. To determine your BMI, divide
your weight in kilograms by the square of height in
meters:

Weight (in kg)

Height (in meters)$^{2.}$

In general, those whom are considered obese are at
higher risk of having fertility challenges.[20] In a review
of 30 studies that included 115,158 men, researchers
found the following results:

- Obesity was associated with more incidence of sperm with DNA fragmentation and abnormal shape (among other sperm-related issues).

- The rate of live births per cycle of ART (assisted reproduction technology) for obese men was reduced compared with men who were not considered obese.

- There was a 10% absolute risk increase of pregnancy that resulted in miscarriage.[21]

Present data consistently show that obesity is associated with reduced reproductive efficiency in men.[22, 23, 24] It is best to maintain a healthy weight not only to support your fertility, but also to set the stage for a healthy life for years to come. (You could seek guidance from a registered dietitian if you would like support for safe, effective weight loss.)

5 MEDITERRANEAN DIET

There are many "diets" that people choose to follow for various reasons. Perusing the internet, one will find suggestions to follow diets such as keto, paleo, and gluten-free to enhance fertility. Although some may see success when following these diets, there is not enough scientific evidence for me to recommend any of these to my clients. The diet that currently appears to have the strongest research-based correlation to enhanced male fertility is the Mediterranean diet.

Adherence to the Mediterranean diet is significantly associated with higher sperm concentration, total sperm count and sperm motility. Dietary patterns characterized by high intakes of fruits, vegetables, whole grains, fish and low intake of meat are associated with better semen quality.[25]

Researchers in Greece evaluated this concept. They assessed dietary intake and its relationship to semen quality. They found that men who did not incorporate many aspects of the Mediterranean diet had an approximately 2.6 times higher likelihood of having abnormal sperm concentration, total sperm count and motility, compared to men who ate more in line with the Mediterranean diet principles.[25]

In another study, men who ate a Mediterranean diet were compared with men who ate a Western diet (high processed meats, fried foods, snacks). The results echoed the results of other studies evaluating the Mediterranean diet and the relation to male fertility. The Mediterranean diet was positively related to sperm count. The researchers also found that men who were obese and followed a Western style diet had a lower sperm count.[26]

Regarding diet and its relationship with assisted reproductive technology outcomes like in-vitro fertilization, a study conducted in the Netherlands showed that couples following the Mediterranean diet during preconception had a higher probability of having a successful IVF cycle and becoming pregnant.[27] Although this sample size used was small and this research was conducted almost 10 years ago, the results provided insight for those undergoing IVF. What Is the "Mediterranean" Diet?

A Mediterranean diet is a general term for the diet followed my many people who live near the Mediterranean Sea. There are slight variations, but for medical purposes, certain guidelines remain consistent. As mentioned above, those that follow a Mediterranean diet may have more positive fertility-related symptoms.

Below are the basic principles of the Mediterranean diet:

- high consumption of fruits, vegetables, whole-grains, beans, nuts and seeds
- olive oil is predominantly used (an important monounsaturated fat source)
- fish and seafood are consumed at least two times a week
- dairy products and poultry are consumed in low to moderate amounts

- eggs are consumed zero to four times a week
- wine is consumed in low/moderate amounts
- red meat and sweets are rarely eaten[28, 29]

In 1993, Oldways, a nonprofit food and nutrition education organization with a mission to inspire healthy eating through cultural food traditions and lifestyles, created the Mediterranean Diet Pyramid – in partnership with the Harvard School of Public Health and the WHO – as an alternative to the USDA's original food pyramid. (See illustration.)

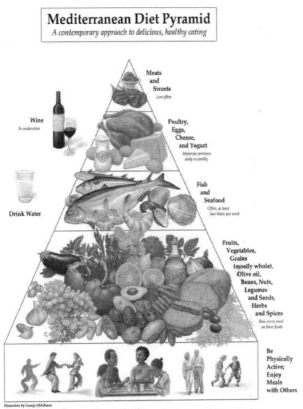

(https://oldwayspt.org/traditional-diets/mediterranean-diet. Accessed October 10, 2018. Used with permission)

MEAT

Meat is not forbidden on this diet, but eaten in moderation. Processed meats are not included, which is consistent with separate findings that processed meat intake does not support male fertility.[26, 30, 31] To investigate this theory, researchers examined 155 men who were considered "subfertile". Men with more problematic sperm morphology had a higher intake of processed red meat. Intake of poultry and unprocessed red meats was unrelated to semen quality.[32]

Examples of processed meats to avoid or minimize include bacon, sausage, ham, corned beef, beef jerky, and salami.

In one study evaluating over 200 men's fertility and meat intake, researchers found that the men who ate the most organ meat had lower sperm motility.[33]

Replacing these foods with fresh fish, poultry, nuts, beans, and other fresh sources of protein is one way to align with Mediterranean diet principles.

ORGANIC VS. CONVENTIONAL PRODUCE

If possible, organic fruits and vegetables are preferred over conventionally-grown produce. The consumption of fruit and vegetables with low-to moderate pesticide residues was positively related to sperm counts in young men.[34] However, conventionally grown produce is better than no produce at all. If organic produce is not an option due to cost, availability, or other factors, choose the produce you have available to you.

6 ANTIOXIDANTS

An antioxidant is a component that is found naturally in many foods, particularly many fruits, vegetables, beans, whole grains, and legumes. Free radicals may attack important molecules in the body, resulting in damage, or oxidative stress. Antioxidants protect cells from the damage caused by these free radicals.[36] Free radicals can come from external sources like smoking or pollutants found in places like the air or water. They may also come about naturally during normal bodily processes like exercise.

Oxidative stress has negative effects on sperm, including viability, shape, and function, and consequently reduces male fertility.[37]

While a small amount of oxidative stress is required for normal sperm functioning, too much negatively impacts the quality of sperm and negatively affects their overall fertilizing ability. Oxidative stress has been shown to play a role in sperm production in the following ways. It can:

- attack DNA, lipids, and proteins in sperm
- alter enzymatic systems
- cause cell death
- cause a decline in the semen measures associated with male infertility[38]

Antioxidants essentially defend the body from oxidative damage, whether it occurs during sperm generation or other functioning of the body. They "neutralize" free radicals, thus preventing them from causing damage.

Antioxidant therapy has been a promising approach to improve the sperm quality and male fertility by reducing oxidative stress.[38]

Examples of foods rich in antioxidants include but are not limited to:

- many fruits and berries
- many vegetables
- whole grains
- dark chocolate
- nuts
- beans
- certain teas such as green and black oolong

Specific examples will follow.

To determine whether antioxidants play a role in male fertility, a literature review was conducted in which reviewers evaluated 35 published studies. Like I have done in this guide, the researchers excluded any animal studies. The researchers found that, among other nutrients, intake of the antioxidants vitamin E, vitamin C, beta-carotene, selenium, zinc, beta-cryptoxanthin and lycopene were related to improved semen quality.[31]

Some examples of food sources of the above antioxidants are below:

Vitamin E	Sunflower seeds, almonds, pistachios, peanut butter, spinach, kiwi, some oil-based salad dressings, walnuts
Vitamin C	Red pepper, orange, grapefruit, kiwi, broccoli, strawberries, baked potato, tomato juice, pears
Beta-Carotene	Sweet potato, carrots, tomato juice, pumpkin, broccoli (many vegetables with a natural orange or yellow pigment and dark leafy greens)
Selenium	Brazil nuts, tuna, sardines, beef liver, cottage cheese, shrimp, brown rice, egg
Zinc	Oysters, crab, fortified cereal, baked beans, dark meat chicken, yogurt, chick peas, cashews
Beta-Cryptoxanthin	Tangerines, persimmons, oranges[39]

Lycopene	Tomatoes (canned, fresh, dried), watermelon, papaya, red grapefruits, and guava.[40] Many foods that have a natural red or pink pigment.

[Unless otherwise noted, source: https://ods.od.nih.gov. Accessed October 11, 2018.]

Researchers wanted to learn whether there is a relationship between certain dietary antioxidants (not in supplement form) and semen quality. A cross-sectional study was conducted using 189 university-age American men. Specifically, they were investigating the dietary intake of Vitamins A, C, E and certain carotenoids like beta-carotene.

After a semen collection and analysis was conducted, certain correlations were found. Findings included:

- Carotenoid intake was associated with better sperm motility

- o Beta-carotene and lutein showed the strongest correlation
- Lycopene was related to better sperm morphology[41]

The most regularly eaten foods that accounted for the largest percentage of antioxidants:

- tomato soup, tomato juice, tomato-based salsa, ketchup and fresh tomatoes accounted for 98% of lycopene intake
- carrots, lettuce and spinach accounted for 59% of beta-carotene intake
- spinach and lettuce accounted for 56% of lutein intake[41]

Another study confirmed the effects of tomato juice consumption and its effect on male infertility. This study demonstrated a positive relationship between male consumption of tomato juice and sperm motility (recall the previous study demonstrated a positive relationship between tomato products and sperm morphology). Studying men who were confirmed to have poor sperm motility, researchers provided men with either one can of tomato juice (with 30 mg lycopene), an antioxidant pill (consisting of 600 mg vitamin C, 200 mg Vitamin E, and 300 mg glutathione)., or nothing (placebo) for 12 weeks. After 12 weeks of following these men, researchers confirmed that there was an improvement in sperm motility for those men who drank tomato juice every day. The antioxidant they provided did not have any effect.[42] It would be interesting to see a study comparing fertility parameters when men drink tomato juice consumption with a lycopene supplement. Maybe one day...

Antioxidants in supplement form

Although I am a "food first" dietitian, meaning that I prefer clients get their nutrients from food sources instead of supplements, many people ask for recommendations on which pills to take when trying to conceive. I recommend dietary interventions as a first-line of defense. If you are going to be taking supplements, the following is information that may help guide you and your health care provider to determine the best supplements to take based on your personal needs.

One research study in particular review evaluated antioxidant intake in nutrient supplement form. The researchers found that in most of the studies, **antioxidant supplementation improved the number, motility, morphology, and sometimes the DNA integrity of sperm.** Antioxidant supplements, especially a combination of antioxidants such as vitamin C, vitamin E, and Coenzyme Q10, intake effectively improved semen parameters in infertile men.[43]

One antioxidant in particular, **zinc**, was studied extensively by researchers in a review conducted in 2018. Zinc (Zn) is the second most abundant trace element in humans, but it can't be stored in the body, thus regular dietary intake is required.

Zinc is essential for male fertility.[44] It has many unique properties in males. It acts as a hormone balancer and may increase testosterone levels.[45] It also acts as an antibacterial agent in men's urinary tract.

Zinc deficiency has been shown to hinder creation of new sperm and plays a role in the development of sperm abnormalities. This is one reason why zinc is often included in male fertility supplements.

Coenzyme Q10 (CoQ10) supplementation is less clear cut. It has been shown to improve total sperm motility and sperm count in some studies, while other studies showed no effect with supplementation. Although there is no standard dose, studies have supported supplementation from 100 mg/day to 300 mg/day.[18,46] However, one study indicated that consumption of CoQ10 from food sources does not have an effect on sperm parameters.[47]

Folate is a B vitamin and antioxidant that helps make DNA and red blood cells in the body and may play a role in male fertility. Folate is the active form of the vitamin and is found in many foods like leafy vegetables, beets, and nuts.

Folic acid is the synthetic form of folate. It is found in a majority of supplements and fortified foods. Folic acid needs to be converted to active folate in the body. Some people are unable to metabolize folic acid properly. Un-metabolized folic acid may be found in people's bloodstreams and may be a cause for concern if taken in high doses.[68] Some studies have linked unmetabolized folic acid with increased cancer risk and undetected vitamin B12 deficiency.[69, 70, 71]

You can have your health care provider help you determine whether you have a methylenetetrahydrofolate reductase (MTHFR) mutation, which would prevent your body from converting folic acid into the active folate in the body. To err on the side of caution, I recommend choosing folate supplements instead of folic acid if supplementation is being explored.

Sources of dietary folate include:

- Avocado
- Spinach

- Black-eyed peas
- Romaine lettuce
- Beets

If a client needs or wishes to supplement his diet, I recommend choosing a supplement that contains the active folate instead of the synthetic folic acid. Active folate may be labeled as L-methylfolate and may be more expensive to purchase.

Although some health care providers and online sources recommend folic acid supplementation for men who are having fertility challenges, there are not enough recent, well-designed studies conducted on humans for me to personally recommend them to men proactively. Incorporating folate-rich foods into your diet is a great way to reap general health benefits of folate, so they are worth considering.

If a man wishes to explore antioxidant supplementation, there is no standard proven dose of each micronutrient to support fertility; in 2018 dosages were recommended based on results from several clinical trials. The trials had to cover basic semen parameters, advanced sperm function tests, assisted reproduction technology outcomes, or live birth rates to be included. Only studies conducted on humans were included.[18]

Please note that these doses are not personal recommendations, and any supplementation should be discussed with your health care provider before consideration.

The most commonly investigated compounds and their doses were as follows:

Vitamin E (400 mg),

Vitamin C (500–1000 mg),

Carnitines (500–1000 mg),

N-acetyl cysteine (NAC; 600 mg),

Co-enzyme Q10(CoQ10; 100–300 mg),

Zinc (25–400 mg),

Selenium (Se) (200 μg),

Folic Acid (0.5 mg), and

Lycopene (6–8 mg)[18]

Because antioxidant treatment has encouraged researchers and medical professionals, proposed antioxidants for various fertility issues based on available evidence are listed below based on a paper published in 2018 by Majzoub and Agarwal.[18]

TABLE 1

Proposed supplemental regimens for low sperm count (oligozoospermia)
Vitamin E (300 mg)
Vitamin E (180 mg), Vitamin A (30 mg) and essential fatty acids or NAC (600 mg)
NAC (600 mg)
L-Carnitine (2 gm)
Coenzyme Q10 (300 mg)
NAC (600 mg) and selenium (200 mcg)
Folic acid (5 mg) and zinc (66 mg)
Lycopene (2 mg)

TABLE 2

Proposed supplemental regimens for reduced sperm motility (Asthenozoospermia)
Vitamin E (400 mg) + selenium (200 µg)
Zinc (400 mg), vitamin E (20 mg) and vitamin C (10 mg)
L-Carnitine (2 g) and L-Acetyl Carnitine (1 g)
CoQ10 (300 mg)
NAC (600 mg)
NAC (600 mg) and selenium (200 µg)
Lycopene (2 mg)

TABLE 3

Proposed supplemental regimens for abnormal sperm shape (Teratozoospermia)
Vitamin E (400 mg) + selenium (200 μg)
NAC (600 mg) and selenium (200 μg)
Zinc (400 mg), vitamin E (20 mg) and vitamin C (10 mg)
Lycopene (8 mg)

TABLE 4

Proposed supplemental regimens for improved Assisted Reproductive Technology rates
Vitamin E (200 mg daily)
Lycopene (6 mg), vitamin E (400 IU), vitamin C (100 mg), zinc (25 mg), selenium (26 g), folate (0.5 mg) and garlic (1 g)
Vitamin E (600 mg)
Vitamin C (1 g) + vitamin E (1 g)

Majzoub A, Agarwal A. Systematic review of antioxidant typles and doses in male infertility: Benefits of semen parameters, advanced sperm function, assisted reproduction and live birth rate. *Arab J Urol.* 2018;16(1):113-124.

The authors mention that further studies are needed to identify the optimal antioxidant regimen that can be used safely and efficiently in clinical practice.[18]

A "mini review" was conducted by the same researchers (along with a third author) to assess antioxidant therapy and the effect on sperm DNA fragmentation. The findings are found in Table 5:[48]

TABLE 5

Proposed supplemental regimens for sperm DNA Fragmentation
Vitamin C (100 mg), E (400 IU), Selenium (26 ìg), Zinc (25 mg), folic acid (0.5 mg) and garlic (1 mg)
Beta-carotene (18 mg), vitamins C (400 mg), E (400 mg), Zn (500 µmol) and Selenium (1 µmol)
Vitamins C (200 mg), E (200 mg), glutathione (400 mg)

Any supplementation should be discussed with your health care provider before adding any pills to your daily regimen. My recommendations typically include encouraging clients to incorporate more antioxidants into their diet before considering supplements.

7 TRANS-FATS

Trans fatty acids (trans-fats) are not naturally-occurring in food, and some studies have shown that they can have negative effects on human health. They are created by adding hydrogen to liquid vegetable oils to make them more solid. The primary dietary source for trans fats in processed food is partially hydrogenated oils. Sources of trans fats include margarines, many baked goods that are shelf-stable for a long time (like the pre-packaged cinnamon rolls you find at the gas station), some frozen pizzas, many fried foods, and some crackers. Trans-fat content is now listed on food labels in the United States. Thankfully, many food companies are moving away from using trans-fats in the foods they manufacture.

All fats are not created equal. **Researchers have stated that not only can they have a negative effect on overall health, there is a negative relationship between trans-fat intake and male fertility parameters.**

One study confirmed that trans-fat intake was related to sperm count. After analyzing the diet of 209 men and their sperm samples, the researchers found a negative relationship between trans-fat intake and sperm count. The higher the trans-fat intake, the lower the man's sperm count.[49]

Many studies have been conducted regarding trans-fat intake and male fertility. In 2018, researchers compiled data from these studies and wrote a review article. After reviewing data over 10 years (2007-2017), they concluded that the more trans-fats men consumed, the lower their sperm concentration and sperm counts.[50]

Some steps to reduce trans fats in your diet include:

- Choose English muffins instead of biscuits.
- Skip the frosting on desserts like cupcakes and cookies.
- Avoid movie popcorn unless the theater specifies that their popcorn is trans-fat free. Avoid microwavable popcorn bags, and pop your kernels yourself.
- Ensure that any French fries you are ordering are not fried in partially hydrogenated vegetable oil. Bake fries instead of frying them at home.
- Do not cook with lard. Choose oils like olive oil when cooking

8 OMEGA-3 FATTY ACIDS/SEAFOOD/NUTS

Omega-3 fatty acids are essential fatty acids, meaning that your body cannot make them, but needs them for proper functioning, so they need to be consumed either though diet or supplements. There are three omega-3 fatty acids:

- Alpha-linolenic acid (ALA)
- Eicosapentaenoic acid (EPA), and
- Docosahexaenoic acid (DHA)

Consumption of omega-3 fatty acids has declined over the years as processed foods and the use of certain oils with low or no omega-3s has increased in American diets.[51]

According to a position paper by the Academy of

Nutrition and Dietetics, expert panels recommend a daily intake of DHA and EPA within the range of 250-500 mg/day for healthy adults. They also recommend 0.6%-1.2% of daily fat intake in the form of ALA.[52]

Although there is promising research on the benefits of certain omega 3 fatty acids and various general aspects of human health, unfortunately, extensive clinical trials regarding male fertility are lacking. What is known is that dietary fatty acids influence sperm fatty acid profiles and omega-3 fatty acids seem particularly influential. For example, higher levels of DHA are concentrated on the human sperm's head vs. other parts of the sperm's "body".

To determine whether there is a correlation between dietary fats and semen quality parameters, fatty acid levels of sperm from 99 mostly Caucasian men were analyzed. It is important to note that 71% of these men were considered overweight or obese. The researchers found that higher intake of omega-3 fatty acids was related to a more favorable sperm morphology. They also found that high intake of saturated fats was associated with worse sperm concentration.[53]

Another study conducted in Spain evaluated intake of different fats and their effect on male fertility. The authors concluded that the consumption of omega-3 fatty acids were positively related to testicular volume.[54]

One 2018 meta-analysis, in particular, reviewed all of the literature available. A meta-analysis is a detailed review of studies that were conducted previously. The results of this meta-analysis found that men who took DHA and EPA supplements of varying dosages showed improvement in sperm motility and concentration of DHA in seminal plasma (the fluid medium in semen that suspends the sperm).[55]

Generally, a minimum consumption of 250– 500 mg/day of combined EPA + DHA is recommended for proper functioning for all healthy adults---men and women. The exact quantity of DHA and EPA for men interested in boosting fertility is unfortunately not established.

Sources of Omega-3 Fatty Acids

DHA and EPA omega-3 fatty acids are found in

foods such as fish and seafood, algae, and certain egg yolks.[56] ALA omega-3 fatty acid is found mainly in plant oils such as flaxseed and walnuts. Omega-3 fatty acids offer health benefits to the human body including a potential fertility benefit.

DHA/EPA

A recent study examined 501 couples trying to conceive. The researchers found that couples who consumed eight or more servings of seafood per menstrual cycle (typically 28 days) required less time to achieve pregnancy compared with couples who ate only one or fewer servings per menstrual cycle. Recall that many seafood choices are rich in DHA and EPA omega-3 fatty acids. Couples who both consumed eight or more servings of seafood *per week* showed even more success, and couples where both partners consumed greater than either servings of seafood per menstrual cycle saw even more success![57] This study does not indicate whether taking omega-3 fatty acid supplements would offer the same benefit. There is a possibility that these results were due to other features of seafood rather than their omega-3 content (like being a protein source low in saturated fat or being high in certain other nutrients). Regardless, seafood consumption has little downside and should be considered when couples are trying to conceive.

During a prospective investigation of 155 infertile men, researchers found that fish intake was related to improved fertility parameters. Specifically, they found:

- sperm count was strongest for intake of dark meat fish like salmon and tuna
- sperm morphology was related most strongly with intake of white meat fish like cod and halibut (but was observed for intake of dark meat fish as well)
- fish intake was related to higher sperm count and more morphologically "normal" sperm[32]

Some people have valid concerns about mercury in some fish, and it is possible to find lower-mercury containing fish and seafood to add to your diet. The Natural Resources Defense Council and the United States Environmental Protection Agency offers an up-to-date chart detailing the mercury levels in a variety of fish and seafood choices.

Popular low-mercury choices that I suggest in my practice are salmon, shrimp, flounder, and oysters. Shark, swordfish king mackerel, and tilefish are examples of fish that are considered to have high levels of mercury.

It is important to note that men should not avoid fish or seafood simply due to the concern of mercury exposure. One study evaluated men's mercury levels via hair samples and fertility parameters. One would assume that if a man's hair has higher amounts of mercury, he consumes a significant amount of fish and seafood (since the general population exposure to mercury is due to consumption of contaminated fish).

The researchers found that the men with the highest concentration of mercury also had the best fertility parameters (sperm concentration, total sperm count, and progressive motility). The researches attribute this to the increased fish/seafood intake that outweighs the downside of consuming mercury. Again, it is better to avoid consuming large amounts of mercury, but the benefit of consuming mercury via fish/seafood appears to outweigh the risk of eating this type of food.[58]

Alpha-Linonenic Acid (ALA)

Alpha-linonenic acid (ALA) is a type of omega-3 fatty acid that is found in plants. It is another fatty acid that has been explored in the world of male fertility, although not as extensively as DHA and EPA omega-3s. Certain nuts and seeds are excellent sources of

ALA omega-3 fatty acids, as well as other nutrients like folate, plant-based protein, antioxidants, and fiber. Researchers tried to answer the question: "Can a continual consumption of a mixture of nuts improve the semen quality parameters and the sperm functionality in healthy individuals?"

Men were either given a nut-free Western-style diet, or a Western-style diet supplemented with 60 grams/day of a mix of almonds, hazelnuts, and walnuts (equivalent to approximately 2 handfuls a day). The authors concluded that including nuts in a regular diet significantly improved men's sperm parameters. Men who ate nuts daily saw a 16 percent increase in sperm count along with improvements in sperm vitality, motility, shape, and size. They also observed a reduction in damaging DNA fragmentation.[59] (This study was funded by the International Nut and Dried Food Council-FYI.)

This study did not include men who were diagnosed with infertility, so the results may not apply to everyone. Additionally, it is unknown if it is the omega-3 content, other nutrient content, or a combination that played a role in these results. Either way, eating nuts are a healthy addition to most people's diets. They are a great snack, easy to add to meals, and provide plant-based protein. Adding 60 grams (approximately 2 handfuls) of mixed nuts per day (as a replacement for other proteins or snacks, if you're watching calorie and nutrition intake) is a practice that can be easily maintained.

Other researchers focused on walnuts, specifically, as a whole food that contains not only essential fatty acids but also antioxidants, and how they might influence sperm development and function. They found that 75 grams of walnuts per day for 12 weeks improved sperm vitality, motility, and morphology (in a group of healthy, young men who consumed a Western-style diet).[60]

Incorporating low-mercury fish and seafood as well as certain nuts into your diet is a simple modification that may support not only your fertility, but also other aspects of your health. If you're considering omega-3 supplementation, I encourage you to ensure your choice is free of contaminants and as pure as possible. Seeking guidance from a registered dietitian can help you make a safe choice.

9 VITAMIN D

Vitamin D is a hot topic these days. It is a fat-soluble vitamin that gets converted into a hormone in the body. It is found in some foods and can also be converted through skin from UV light from the sun.

Vitamin D plays many roles in the human body, and some theorize that a deficiency may influence infertility. In general, the recommended dietary allowance of Vitamin D for adult men under the age of 70 years old is 600 IU/day[61], although some argue it should be higher due to the prevalence of Vitamin D deficiency in the United States. Some say that more than 40 percent of the U.S. population is vitamin D deficient.[62] One contributing factor to this issue is the modern lifestyle most of us live, with limited skin exposure to sunlight and, thus, limited exposure to the UV light.

The role of vitamin D in hormone production and sperm creation has been investigated in both animals and humans. Experimental studies support a beneficial effect of vitamin D on male fertility by playing a role in hormone production and by improving sperm parameters. [23, 31, 63]

Clinical studies in humans regarding Vitamin D and fertility have been controversial and more research is needed. Some studies have demonstrated a positive effect of Vitamin D intake on semen quality and motility according to a literature review.[64] Conversely, a study conducted with men specifically undergoing IVF demonstrated no correlation between vitamin D status and any fertility variables (motility, count, or morphology).[65]

In regard to the studies that suggest the positive effect of Vitamin D on male fertility, it is important to note that vitamin D does not appear to exert an important role in human fertility *in the absence of deficiency*.[66] In other words, if a man already has adequate Vitamin D levels, supplementation will not likely provide a benefit.

Determining whether there is a true vitamin D deficiency requires a blood test. It is relatively inexpensive and easily accessible. If a man is diagnosed with a vitamin D deficiency, in general, it is a good idea to ensure adequate vitamin D intake to replenish levels for many reasons beyond fertility. If supplementation is being considered, the medical community generally recommends taking the D3 form (not the D2 form).

Some dietary sources of Vitamin D include:

- fatty fish like salmon and tuna
- egg yolks
- dairy drinks and dairy-alternative drinks fortified with Vitamin D
- certain mushrooms
- Vitamin D-fortified orange juice and yogurt[67]

Additionally, direct exposure of skin to sunlight allows Vitamin D to naturally be converted in the body.

LAUREN MANAKER MS, RDN, LD, CLEC

10 DAIRY

Dairy has become a polarizing topic in the nutrition world. As a registered dietitian, I am a fan of dairy foods. They can be a positive addition to a healthy diet and provide an array of nutrients for the body including protein, calcium, phosphorus, and Vitamin D. Dairy foods are probably best-known to support healthy bones.

If a client is not a dairy eater or drinker, I don't try to sway him from his preference. However, if a client normally consumes dairy products, I share current evidence on how these foods may affect male fertility.

When dairy intake and its relationship to general male fertility is evaluated, evidence suggests that men should stick with the low-fat dairy products and skim milk.[23, 31] Though data suggests that men's dairy intake does *not* affect IVF outcomes.[34] In a focused study, when evaluating past or current smokers, one study found that cheese intake reduces sperm concentration and motility, but low-fat milk intake was related to higher sperm concentration (among smokers and non-smokers).[72]

Some studies may suggest that dairy choice does not make a difference, however most studies I have come across support the intake of low-fat or skim dairy foods for men.

If you are already consuming dairy foods, if you already choose low-fat or skim milk options, you're on the right track. If not, these dairy options may be a lifestyle change to consider trying.

11 SOY

Soy foods include tofu, edamame, and certain meat alternatives. Soy contains phytoestrogens, or components that act in the body like the hormone estrogen. Some men hear the words "natural estrogen" and immediately assume they should stay away from those foods. One of the best-designed studies to support this theory was conducted over a decade ago, studying almost 100 men as subjects. After analyzing soy intake and its relationship to male fertility parameters, the researchers found that men who consumed the most soy in their diet had significantly fewer sperm compared with men who did not consume soy. Soy food and soy isoflavone intake were unrelated to sperm motility, sperm morphology or ejaculate volume.[73]

One study conducted in 2015 with a sample size of 184 men disproves that theory. Although some studies suggest that consumption of soy foods may affect male hormone levels, it may not affect the end-goal of pregnancy, at least when undergoing IVF. The researchers found that soy food intake was unrelated to fertilization rates, the proportions of poor-quality embryos, accelerated or slow embryo cleavage rate, and implantation, clinical pregnancy, and live birth.[74]

In a review article in which the authors conducted a comprehensive assessment of the available literature, the authors state that the evidence on male fertility and soy intake is conflicting; some studies demonstrated a negative impact caused by soy consumption and others showed no effect.[75]

In the case of soy, I recommend a moderate consumption if a man typically enjoys these foods since as mentioned previously the research is inconclusive. I would not make a point to incorporate these foods, but total elimination does not appear to be necessary.

12 ALCOHOL

The association between alcohol intake
and male reproductive function is still controversial.[76]
I will highlight some studies that have been
conducted on the topic, although this is not
comprehensive.

In one study conducted in Italy with couples
struggling with infertility, the men's alcohol
consumption was assessed (as well as other factors).
The men who participated in the study had an average
age being 39 years old. Surprisingly, moderate alcohol
intake was positively associated with semen quality!
Men who drank fewer than three servings of alcohol
per week had lower semen volume than "moderate
"drinkers. The authors define moderate drinkers as
those who drink 4 to 7 drinks of alcohol per week
containing 12.5 g of ethanol (125 mL wine or 330 mL
beer or 30 mL spirits).[76] This doesn't mean you

should go out and guzzle a keg of beer a day, but it does imply that moderate drinking may not be seriously harmful to male fertility.

In a review paper published in 2018, the researchers confirmed the conflicting data on alcohol intake when trying to conceive.[20] On one hand, they report results from a meta-analysis involving 29,914 men in which there was no significant relationship between alcohol intake and sperm parameters.[77]

On the other hand, a study evaluating chronic drinkers and fertility parameters suggests a negative relationship. Researchers classified chronic drinkers as those who drank a minimum of 180 mL of either brandy or whisky per day for a minimum of 5 days per week for ≥1 year. Researchers compared fertility parameters of chronic drinkers with men who did not drink chronically. Hormones were affected, including a reduction in testosterone in the men who were labeled "chronic drinkers". Semen volume, sperm count, motility, and number of morphologically normal sperm were significantly decreased.[78]

Some men pursuing Assisted Reproduction Technology (ART) undergo a process called intracytoplasmic sperm injection (ICSI). During this process, sperm is directly injected into an egg in a lab, typically by an embryologist.

For couples undergoing ICSI, fertilization rate was reduced in men who consumed alcohol in one study. The authors of the study recommend that men undergoing IVF with ICSI refrain from alcohol.[79]

However, for men not undergoing IVF with ICSI, alcohol consumption is one factor that is not as clear. The evidence regarding male alcohol consumption and its effect on fertility is inconclusive, and more research is needed to make a definitive recommendation.

Excessive alcohol intake is not recommended. In my opinion, having a maximum of one alcoholic drink per day would likely not have a large effect on male fertility.

13 CAFFEINE

According to Bill Hicks, an American comedian, "There are essentially only two drugs that Western civilization tolerates: Caffeine from Monday to Friday to energize you enough to make you a productive member of society, and alcohol from Friday to Monday to keep you too stupid to figure out the prison that you are living in." After discussing alcohol, the logical next topic would have to be caffeine intake!

Like alcohol, evidence related to caffeine's influence on male fertility is conflicting.

Caffeine intake may impair male reproductive function possibly through sperm DNA damage.[20] A meta-analysis of this topic was conducted in 2017. A meta-analysis is a detailed review of studies that were conducted previously. In this meta-analysis, 28 papers were evaluated, including in total 19,967 men. The authors concluded the following:

- Measures of semen quality did not seem affected by caffeine intake from coffee, tea, and cocoa drinks, in most studies.

- A negative effect of caffeine-containing soft drinks on semen volume, count, and concentration was seen.

- DNA breaks in sperm were seen with caffeine consumption, but not with other markers of DNA damage.

- Male coffee drinking was associated with requiring a longer time to achieve successful pregnancy in some, but not all, studies[80]

For couples undergoing IVF, male intake of caffeine and pregnancy outcomes is also conflicting. In one recent study evaluating caffeine intake and rates of pregnancy for couples undergoing IVF, male caffeine intake was negatively related to live birth.[81] However, in another study, results indicated that a moderate caffeine intake in the year prior to the IVF procedure was not associated with negative IVF outcomes.[82]

Although study results are conflicting, experts have stated that a high level of caffeine intake by the male has a negative influence on the chance of pregnancy or fertilization rates in their partners.[31]

As a registered dietitian, **I typically recommend that men refrain from drinking sugary sodas that contain caffeine when trying to conceive, regardless of whether they are undergoing assisted reproductive technology (ART).** Soda consumption has not been associated with any fertility benefit, and there are plenty of other alternative beverages that men can enjoy. Water is a more beneficial hydration source.

In terms of other caffeine sources, **it does not appear that men need to be as cautious as women do when trying to enhance fertility. Excessive caffeine intake is likely not the best choice when trying to conceive, but moderate or low intake seems not to have a negative impact.** Unfortunately, the term "excessive" is different depending on the individual since genetics plays a role in individual variability in caffeine consumption and in the direct effects of caffeine.

To be on the safe side, be cautious of how many caffeine-containing beverages you are consuming in a day (such as coffee, teas, matchas, chocolate, energy drinks). One or two servings should be fine depending on the individual. If you are a caffeine addict (like many people are), try to scale down by swapping one coffee with a decaffeinated beverage. Over time, increase the ratio of decaf beverages for caffeinated drinks.

14 LIFESTYLE ISSUES
EXERCISE/SLEEP/STRESS

EXERCISE

"If we could give every individual the right amount of nourishment and exercise, not too little and not too much, we would have found the safest way to health." ~Hippocrates

Keeping one's body healthy takes a balance of diet and exercise. There is evidence mounting that the right amount of exercise is linked to enhanced male fertility.

Exercise training has been shown to strengthen antioxidant defenses.[83]

Researchers have stated that moderate intensity aerobic exercise results in the healthiest sperm, even when compared with men who perform intense exercise more frequently.[84]

Resistance exercise training has been shown to improve pregnancy rates and sperm parameters in infertile patients.[85]

Intense physical activity may negatively affect the semen concentration, as well as the number of motile and morphologically normal sperm. Training at higher intensities and with increased loads seems to be associated with negative changes in semen quality. However, in recreational or moderate athletes, exercise has either a positive or neutral effect on semen parameters.[86]

Elevated scrotal temperatures related to motor sports[87] and cycling[88] may play a role in male fertility impairment as well. Cycling has been associated with abnormal sperm morphology and reduced motility.[89, 90]

Like most things, too much of a good thing can be

bad. Exercise is a wonderful thing to incorporate into your life if you are trying to conceive, but too much intensity could have negative effects. Stick with 30 to 45 minutes of exercise with moderate intensity and without potential for elevated scrotal temperature at least 3 times a week along with some resistance training, and you should be in good shape!

SLEEP

Sleep is the golden thread that ties our health and our bodies together ~ Thomas Deekkar

Getting adequate sleep appears to be a challenge in modern society. Unfortunately, not getting enough sleep can have negative effects on your health including (you guessed it) male fertility.

A study published in 2017 demonstrated a relationship between sleep and sperm counts. After evaluating 980 men, the researchers found that sperm count and their survival rates were lower in those who went to bed late (after midnight) and got little sleep (fewer than 6 hours). The researchers suspect late bedtimes and little sleep trigger the increase of antisperm antibody, a protein produced by the immune system, which can destroy healthy sperm.[91] Interestingly, the authors also suggest that sleeping more than nine hours a night had a negative effect on male fertility parameters. Between 7 and 8 hours of sleep is ideal.

Another study evaluated 1,176 men who were attempting to conceive for up to six months. Results confirmed that less than six hours of sleep resulted in lower pregnancy success rates.[92]

Currently, there are still limited data about how men's sleeping patterns influence fertility. However, a common finding is **men should aim for seven to eight hours of sleep every evening to enhance fertility, especially if sperm count is an issue**.

STRESS

"The greatest weapon against stress is our ability to choose one thought over another." ~ *William James*

Well-meaning people give the old advice of "relaxing" for pregnancy to occur. I personally thought that was one of the most annoying tidbits I used to hear when

I was trying to conceive. I HATE to be "that person", but it is true. Stress has been shown to be related to male fertility in a negative way.[110, 111]

A diagnosis of infertility can be stressful on its own. Compound it with the daily stresses of work and responsibilities, and stress can truly start affecting your health.

Finding healthy methods to cope with stress is important for fertility and overall well-being. It has to be a priority for you and your partner to carve out some time to do what you need to do to relieve some stress in your life when trying to conceive.

LAUREN MANAKER MS, RDN, LD, CLEC

15 CIGARETTE SMOKING

It is in your best interest to quit smoking if trying to conceive.[93] Cigarette smoking is a known potential risk factor for decreased male fertility. Items such as nicotine, tar, and heavy metals found in cigarettes may negatively affect sperm function and ultimately compromise male fertility.[20]

The American Society of Reproductive Medicine (ASRM) produced an updated committee opinion about smoking's relationship with infertility. "Reductions in sperm density, motility, antioxidant activity, and a possible adverse effect on morphology have been demonstrated" from cigarette smoke (including passive inhalation) according to the ASRM.[94] Chewing tobacco has also demonstrated negative effects on semen parameters.[95]

Bottom line, smoking cigarettes does not support male fertility.

16 MARIJUANA USE

Marijuana use has not been shown to enhance fertility. It is a common refrain that marijuana, or cannabis, is "natural" and harmless. Although this drug has been shown to have a positive effect for some medical issues, it has not been confirmed to enhance fertility in men. Surprisingly, very few studies have explored the direct effect of marijuana on male fertility. This can mainly be ascribed to legislation and ethical considerations making it very difficult to pursue in live human studies.[96]

In one study, researchers found that men who smoked cannabis more than once a week had a 28% lower sperm concentration than those who had not used cannabis. Sperm concentration and total sperm count was lower when marijuana was used in combination with other recreational drugs including amphetamine, cocaine, and/or ecstasy.[97]

Cannabidiol, or CBD, has become a popular supplement in oil form in recent years. Although clinical trials regarding male fertility factors and CBD oil use do not exist, a study using mice was published in late 2018. When comparing mice who were provided with CBD oil vs. placebo, the researchers found that the mice who ingested CBD had a 30% reduction in fertility rate.[98]

Although some studies suggest that marijuana use does not have any significant effect on male fertility,[99, 100] most studies define a negative impact on fertility potential.[101]

I have not personally come across any human studies showing that cannabis *enhances* men's success with conception. Although the benefit of marijuana cessation on recovery is uncertain,[102] I still recommend abstaining from using it recreationally.

17 SCROTAL TEMPERATURE UNDERGARMENT CHOICES, ELECTRONICS

BOXERS VS. BRIEFS

After all of the serious issues covered so far, it's good to get a chuckle out of this topic. Silly as the boxer vs briefs question may seem, I want to address the debate.

Some people feel comfortable wearing tight briefs-style underwear (and Speedo-like bathing suits or bike shorts), which can retain heat. On the other side of the fence are those who only wear boxer shorts, which allow more air flow.

The controversy rests on whether it's "hot" to be hot down below or actually a bad idea for conception. Therefore, a scientific review of your skivvies makes sense.

It was determined that it is critical to maintain a testicular temperature at a level lower than that of the body core as increased testicular temperature has a negative effect on the process of making sperm.[20]

A very recent and well-designed study was conducted in 2018 to get to the "bottom" of the controversy. In total, 656 men were evaluated for type of underwear worn and any correlation with sperm parameters. The results indicate that the men who wore boxer shorts had a 25% higher sperm concentration vs. men who did not wear boxer shorts. They also had a 17% higher total sperm count vs. the men who did not wear boxer shorts.[103] Although there are a lot of variables to this study, it is a step in the right direction to determine whether underwear type makes a difference!

The bottom line (figuratively speaking…) is that staying away from tight underwear is a wise choice, and relatedly, it suggested that men avoid other situations that may elevate scrotal temperatures (like wearing tight pants or soaking in a very hot tub).

LAPTOP/CELLPHONE USE

One small detail to add (as I am typing this with my computer on my lap): when researchers evaluated the effect of exposing men to electromagnetic radiation emitted by wi-fi-enabled laptops, they found that sperm motility was negatively affected.[104] The sample size was small, and this study was only conducted on one specific population. To be on the safe side, don't type away for hours with your laptop resting on your lap. Use your desk or a pillow instead!

Cell phone use is also associated with symptoms of infertility. In one study, the amount of time spent talking on a cell phone was associated with reduced sperm concentrations and sperm count.[105] Another study did not show the same negative effects of talking on a cell phone. Rather, it demonstrated a negative relationship between wireless internet use on a cell phone and sperm count.[106]

A meta-analysis was conducted regarding this topic using ten studies. Exposure to mobile phones was associated with reduced sperm motility and viability.[107] Unfortunately, it appears that mobile phone exposure negatively affects sperm quality. Just one more reason to cut back on that IG addiction…I know easier said than done (trust me-I get it!).

18 HORMONE AND ENDOCRINE DISRUPTORS

"Hormones get no respect. We think of them as the elusive chemicals that make us a bit moody, but these magical little molecules do so much more." ~Susannah Cahalan

Your endocrine system is responsible for releasing hormones in your body. One hormone that your endocrine system is responsible for is testosterone. If testosterone levels are negatively affected, certain consequences like decreased sperm production may ensue.

There are chemicals that are considered "endocrine-disrupting chemicals" (EDCs) or "hormone disruptors" that may disturb your endocrine system, and therefore may affect your fertility. If your endocrine system is disturbed, your fertility may be negatively affected.

Dioxins, polychlorinated biphenyl (PCBs), chlorinated pesticides, brominated flame retardants, bisphenol A (BPA), triclosan, perfluorinated compounds and phthalates are known as endocrine disrupting chemicals. Reduced sperm production as well as congenital abnormalities of male genitalia can be seen in laboratory animals by exposing them to chemicals with endocrine-disrupting effect, and in humans similar effects have been seen following accidental exposures to very high concentrations of these environmental toxins.[108]

In a study evaluating men who were patients of a fertility clinic, the researchers concluded that **concentrations of endocrine-disrupting chemicals are associated with an increased risk of fertility challenges.** The results emphasize the importance of reducing chemicals in the environment in order to safeguard male fertility.[109]

Hormone-disrupting chemicals are unfortunately very

prevalent in many items you may use every day. Depending on the brand, cleaning supplies, personal care items, and even protein powders may be loaded with endocrine disruptors.

Unfortunately, eliminating all hormone-disruptors from your life is nearly impossible.

I recommend starting with one or two changes in your lifestyle, then slowly incorporate more interventions into your life. I would continue this practice even after your partner becomes pregnant. Her exposure to these chemicals may have negative effects to your future child's health, too!

Some simple steps to eliminating hormone-disruptors:

- Avoid heavily fragranced body sprays, lotions, and deodorants unless they are scented with essential oils.
- Do not heat any food in a plastic container or covered with plastic wrap. Store hot food in glass containers.
- Choose fresh, frozen, or dried foods instead of canned foods.

- Cook using stainless steel or cast-iron pans instead of non-stick pans.
- Replace chemically-based cleaning supplies with a mixture of vinegar, water, and baking soda when possible.
- Visit the "Environmental Working Group" website (www.ewg.org) to evaluate how many hormone disruptors are present in the personal care items you currently use. Switch to more "clean" items.

19 RECOMMENDATIONS/CONCLUSIONS

When considering options of how to enhance male fertility, there is very little (if any) downside to incorporating changes like eating more low-mercury seafood, maintaining a healthy weight, or quitting smoking.

For couples having difficulty getting pregnant, the mounting evidence that men's fertility should be focused on just as much as the woman's means that men don't have to be bystanders in the process as much as previously thought. Even incorporating a few modifications from this guide can help you lead an overall healthy life and possibly lead you down a successful path to your pregnancy goals.

Below is a list of dietary and lifestyle modifications that can be made for the most prevalent issues I see in my practice. This list is a starting point, not all encompassing. The previous sections of this guide provide additional dietary and lifestyle modifications with more details.

I recommend making two or three dietary or lifestyle changes at a time, and once they become a part of your lifestyle, you could consider making more. I do not recommend trying to make too many changes at once. The "all or nothing" approach is not sustainable, unless you are at a critically important stage of life or the fertility process and your doctor advises that you need to make drastic changes. You, your partner, and your doctor can decide that together.

LOW SPERM COUNT (Oligozoospermia)

- Adhere to the Mediterranean Diet guidelines.[25, 26] See the section on the Mediterranean diet for specific details and focus on one or two modifications at a time.

- Eat a diet rich in antioxidants. For a list of specific antioxidants that have been studied and supplemented for this condition, refer to Table 1 in the "antioxidants" section of this guide for more details.

- Eat 60 gm (approx. 2 handfuls) of a mixture of almonds, walnuts, and hazelnuts per day.[59]

- Choose drinks other than cola-containing beverages and caffeine-containing soft drinks.[80]

- Choose skim milk instead of whole milk.[72]

- Stop smoking cigarettes.[93]

- Stop taking recreational drugs, including marijuana.[97]

- Avoid endocrine-disrupting items like cans that contain BPA and fragrance-filled body sprays.[109]

- Include dark meat fish into your diet like salmon.[32]

- Ensure between seven and eight hours of sleep a night.[92]

REDUCED SPERM MOTILITY
(Asthenozoospermia)

- Adhere to the Mediterranean Diet guidelines.[25, 26] See the section on the Mediterranean diet for specific details and focus on one or two modifications at a time.

- Eat a diet rich in antioxidants. For a list of specific antioxidants that have been studied and supplemented for this condition, refer to Table 2 in the "antioxidants" section of this guide for more details.

- Eat 60 gm mixed nuts/day (almonds, walnuts, and hazelnuts).[59]

- Ensure you are not deficient in vitamin D. If you are diagnosed with vitamin D deficiency, increase vitamin D intake by consuming foods like egg yolks and fatty fish or consider supplementation with Vitamin D3 if needed.[64]

- Discuss Coenzyme Q10 supplementation with your doctor.[46]

- Consume foods rich in beta carotene and lutein (like egg yolks and carrots)

- Participate in moderately intense exercise.[86]

SPERM MORPHOLOGY/SHAPE ISSUES
(Teratozoospermia)

- Adhere to the Mediterranean Diet guidelines.[25] See the section on the Mediterranean diet for specific details and focus on one or two modifications at a time.

- Eat a diet rich in antioxidants. For a list of specific antioxidants that have been studied and supplemented for this condition, refer to Table 3 in the "antioxidants" section for more details.

- Eat 60 gm mixture of almonds, walnuts, and hazelnuts per day.[59]

- Eat lycopene-rich foods (like tomato-based soups and salsa).[41]

- Maintain a weight that is not considered obese.[21]

- Eliminate cigarette smoking.[20]

- Reduce processed red meat intake.[32]

- Incorporate white meat fish like cod and halibut into your diet.[32]

LOW TESTOSTERONE

- Avoid testosterone replacement therapy without your doctor's consent.[17]

- Avoid endocrine-disrupting items like cans that contain BPA and fragrance-filled body sprays.[109]

- Include zinc-rich foods like oysters, crab, baked beans, and cashews.[16]

- Do not eat soy foods in excess.[74]

- Ensure a Vitamin D deficiency does not exist and consume adequate vitamin D or supplement if necessary.[23]

- Avoid chronic alcohol consumption.[78]

DNA FRAGMENTATION

- Eat 60 gm mixed nuts/day (almonds, walnuts, and hazelnuts).[59]

- Consume caffeine in moderation.[20]

- If obese, gradually lose weight to ensure an ideal BMI.[21]

- Eat a diet rich in antioxidants.[43] If considering supplementation, refer to Table 5 in the "antioxidant" section of this guide for more details.[18]

CONCLUSION

There is no such thing as the "perfect fertility diet," as some research is conflicting, more evidence seems to emerge daily, and more research is still needed.

However, I compiled the best evidence currently available to make navigating the world of infertility a little less overwhelming, and hopefully bring you one step closer to fatherhood.

For further information, email me at NutritionNowCounseling@gmail.com. I am happy to help!

20 REFERENCES

1. Ely D, Hamilton B. Trends in Fertility and Mother's Age at First Birth Among Rural and Metropolitan Counties: United States, 2007–2017. Center for Disease Control and Prevention NCHS Data Brief. 2018(323). https://www.cdc.gov/nchs/data/databriefs/db323-h.pdf. Accessed October 18, 2018.

2. Centers for Disease Control and Prevention. *Infertility* FAQs. Updated April 18, 2018. http://www.cdc.gov/reproductivehealth/infertility. Accessed October 15, 2018.

3. Agarwal A, Mulgund A, Hamada A, Chyatte MR. A unique view on male infertility around the globe. *Reprod Biol Endocrinol.* 2015 Apr 26;13:37. doi: 10.1186/s12958-015-0032-1.

4. Menezo Y, Evenson D, Cohen M, Dale B. Effect of antioxidants on sperm genetic damage. *Adv Exp Med Biol.* 2014;791:173-89. doi: 10.1007/978-1-4614-7783-9_11.

5. National Institute of Health. How common is male infertility, and what are its causes?

Reviewed 12/1/2016.
https://www.nichd.nih.gov/health/topics/m
enshealth/conditioninfo/infertility. Accessed
December 24, 2018.

6. Nassan FL, Chavarro JE, Tanrikut C. Diet
    and men's fertility: does diet affect sperm
    quality? *Fertil Steril.* 2018 Sep;110(4):570-577.
    doi: 10.1016/j.fertnstert.2018.05.025.

7. Barker M, Dombrowski SU, Colbourn T, Fall
    CHD, Kriznik NM, Lawrence WT, et al.,
    Intervention strategies to improve nutrition
    and health behaviours before conception.
    Lancet 2018;391(10132):1853-1864. doi:
    10.1016/S0140-6736(18)30313-1. Epub 2018
    Apr 16.

8. Efremov EA, Kasatonova EV, Mel'nik JI.
    Male Preconception Care. *Urologiia.* 2015 May-
    Jun;(3):97-100, 102-4.

9. Stephenson J, Heslehurst N, Hall
    J, Schoenaker DAJM, Hutchinson J, Cade
    JE, Poston L, Barrett G, Crozier SR, Barker
    M, Kumaran K, Yajnik CS, Baird J, Mishra
    GD. Before
    the beginning: nutrition and lifestyle in the
    preconception period and its importance for
    future health. *Lancet.* 2018 May

5;391(10132):1830-1841. doi: 10.1016/S0140-6736(18)30311-8. Epub 2018 Apr 16.

10. Durairajanayagam D, Rengan A. Sperm Biology from Production to Ejaculation. Unexplained Infertility. In: Schattman G., Esteves S., Agarwal A. (eds) Unexplained Infertility. Springer, New York, NY; 2015.

11. Kumar N, Singh AK. Trends of male factor infertility, an important cause of infertility: A review of literature. *J Hum Reprod Sci.* 2015 Oct-Dec;8(4):191-6. doi: 10.4103/0974-1208.170370.

12. Levine H, Jørgensen N, Martino-Andrade A, Mendiola J, Weksler-Derri D, Mindlis I, Pinotti R, Swan SH. Temporal trends in sperm count: a systematic review and meta-regression analysis. *Hum Reprod Update.* 2017 Nov 1;23(6):646-659. doi: 10.1093/humupd/dmx022.

13. Jarow J, Sigman M, Kolettis PN, Lipshultz LR, McClure D, *et al.* The Optimal Evaluation of the Infertile Male: AUA Best Practice Statement. American Urological Association. 2010. https://www.auanet.org/documents/education/clinical-guidance/Male-infertility-d.pdf. Accessed November 22, 2018.

14. Patel AS, Leong JY, Ramasamy R. Prediction of male infertility by the World Health Organization laboratory manual for assessment of semen analysis: A systematic review. *Arab J Urol.* 2017 Nov 20;16(1):96-102. doi: 10.1016/j.aju.2017.10.005. eCollection 2018 Mar.

15. Docshop. Male factor infertility. Updated Sept 6, 2017. https://www.docshop.com/education/fertility/causes/male. Accessed November 22, 2018.

16. Kothari S, Thompson A, Agarwal A, du Plessis SS. Free radicals: their beneficial and detrimental effects on sperm function. *Indian J Exp Biol.* 2010 May;48(5):425-35.

17. McBride JA, Coward RM. Recovery of spermatogenesis following testosterone replacement therapy or anabolic-androgenicsteroid use. *Asian J Androl.* 2016 May-Jun;18(3):373-80. doi: 10.4103/1008-682X.173938.

18. Majzoub A, Argawal A. Systematic review of antioxidant types and doses in male infertility: Benefits on semen parameters, advanced sperm function, assisted reproduction and

live-birth rate. *Arab J Urol.* 2018 Mar; 16(1): 113–124.

19. Centers for Disease Control and Prevention. Overweight and obesity. Updated August 13, 2018. https://www.cdc.gov/obesity/data/adult.html. Accessed October 16, 2018.

20. Durairajanayagam D. Lifestyle causes of male infertility. *Arab J Urol.* 2018; 16(1): 10–20.

21. Campbell J.M., Lane M., Owens J.A., Bakos H.W. Paternal obesity negatively affects male fertility and assisted reproduction outcomes: a systematic review and meta-analysis. *Reprod Biomed Online.* 2015;31:593–604.

22. Chavarro JE, Schlaff WD. Introduction: Impact of nutrition on reproduction: an overview. *Fertil Steril.* 2018 Sep;110(4):557-559. doi: 10.1016/j.fertnstert.2018.07.023.

23. Silva T, Jesus M, Cagigal C, Silva C. Food with influence in the sexual and reproductive health. *Curr Pharm Biotechnol.* 2018 Sep 25. doi: 10.2174/1389201019666180925140400.

24. Adewoyin M, Ibrahim M, Roszaman R, Isa MLM, Alewi NAM, Rafa AAA, Anuar MNN. Male Infertility: The Effect of Natural Antioxidants and Phytocompounds on

Seminal Oxidative Stress. *Diseases.* 2017 Mar 1;5(1). pii: E9. doi: 10.3390/diseases5010009.

25. Karayiannis D, Kontogianni MD, Mendorou C, Douka L, Mastrominas M, Yiannakouris N. Association between adherence to the Mediterranean diet and semen quality parameters in male partners of couples attempting fertility. Hum Reprod. 2017 Jan;32(1):215-222. Epub 2016 Nov 14.

26. Cutillas-Tolín A, Mínguez-Alarcón L, Mendiola J, López-Espín JJ, Jørgensen N, Navarrete-Muñoz EM, Torres-Cantero AM, Chavarro JE. Mediterranean and western dietary patterns are related to markers of testicular function among healthy men. *Hum Reprod.* 2015 Dec;30(12):2945-55. doi: 10.1093/humrep/dev236. Epub 2015 Sep 25.

27. Vujkovic M, de Vries JH, Lindemans J, Macklon NS, van der Spek PJ, Steegers EA, Steegers-Theunissen RP. The preconception Mediterranean dietary pattern in couples undergoing in vitro fertilization/intracytoplasmic sperm injection treatment increases the chance of pregnancy. *Fertil Steril.* 2010 Nov;94(6):2096-101. doi:

10.1016/j.fertnstert.2009.12.079. Epub 2010 Mar 1.

28. American Heart Association. Mediterranean Diet. Reviewed April 18, 2018. http://www.heart.org/en/healthy-living/healthy-eating/eat-smart/nutrition-basics/mediterranean-diet. Accessed October 16, 2018.

29. Oldways. Mediterranean Diet. https://oldwayspt.org/traditional-diets/mediterranean-diet. Accessed October 16, 2018.

30. Xia W, Chiu YH, Williams PL, Gaskins AJ, Toth TL, Tanrikut C, Hauser R, Chavarro JE. Men's meat intake and treatment outcomes among couples undergoing assisted reproduction. *Fertil Steril.* 2015 Oct;104(4):972-979. doi: 10.1016/j.fertnstert.2015.06.037. Epub 2015 Jul 20.

31. Salas-Huetos A, Bulló M, Salas-Salvadó J. Dietary patterns, foods and nutrients in male fertility parameters and fecundability: a systematic review of observational studies. *Hum Reprod Update.* 2017 Jul 1;23(4):371-389. doi: 10.1093/humupd/dmx006.

32. Afeiche MC, Gaskins AJ, Williams PL, Toth TL, Wright DL, Tanrikut C., *et al.* Processed meat intake is unfavorably and fish intake favorably associated with semen quality indicators among men attending a fertility clinic. *J Nutr.* 2014 Jul;144(7):1091-8. doi: 10.3945/jn.113.190173. Epub 2014 May 21.

33. Maldonado-Cárceles AB, Mínguez-Alarcón L, Mendiola J, Vioque J, Jørgensen N, Árense-Gonzalo JJ, Torres-Cantero AM, Chavarro, J. Meat intake in relation to semen quality and reproductive hormone levels among young men in Spain. *Br J Nutr.* 2018 Dec 18:1-10. doi: 10.1017/S0007114518003458. [Epub ahead of print]

34. Xia W, Chiu YH, Afeiche MC, Williams PL, Ford JB, Tanrikut C, Souter I, Hauser R, Chavarro JE; EARTH study team. Impact of men's dairy intake on assisted reproductive technology outcomes among couples attending a fertility clinic. *Andrology.* 2016 Mar;4(2):277-83. doi: 10.1111/andr.12151. Epub 2016 Jan 29.

35. Lobo V, Patil A, Phatak A, Chandra N. Free radicals, antioxidants and functional foods:

Impact on human health. *Pharmacogn Rev.* 2010 Jul;4(8):118-26.

36. National Cancer Institute. NCI dictionary of cancer terms: antioxidant. https://www.cancer.gov/publications/diction aries/cancer-terms/def/antioxidant. Accessed October 16, 2018.

37. Harlev A, Agarwal A, Gunes SO, Shetty A, du Plessis SS. Smoking and Male Infertility: An Evidence-Based Review. *World J Mens Health.* 2015;33(3):143-60. doi: 10.5534/wjmh.2015.33.3.143. Epub 2015 Dec 23.

38. Sabeti P, Pourmasumi S, Rahiminia T, Akyash F, Talebi AR. Etiologies of sperm oxidative stress. *Int J Reprod Biomed (Yazd).* 2016 Apr;14(4):231-40.

39. Burri BJ. Beta-cryptoxanthin as a source of vitamin A. *J Sci Food Agric.* 2015 Jul;95(9):1786-94. doi: 10.1002/jsfa.6942. Epub 2014 Nov 5.

40. Mozos I, Stoian D, Caraba A, Malainer C, Horbańczuk JO, Atanasov AG. Lycopene and Vascular Health. *Front Pharmacol.* 2018 May 23;9:521. doi: 10.3389/fphar.2018.00521. eCollection 2018.

41. Zareba P, Colaci DS, Afeiche M, Gaskins AJ, Jørgensen N, Mendiola J, Swan SH, Chavarro JE. Semen quality in relation to antioxidant intake in a healthy male population. *Fertil Steril.* 2013 Dec;100(6):1572-9. doi: 10.1016/j.fertnstert.2013.08.032. Epub 2013 Oct 2.

42. Yamamoto Y, Aizawa K, Mieno M, Karamatsu M, Hirano Y, Furui K, *et al.* The effects of tomato juice on male infertility. *Asia Pac J Clin Nutr.* 2017 Jan;26(1):65-71. doi: 10.6133/apjcn.102015.17.

43. Ahmadi S, Bashiri R, Ghadiri-Anari A, Nadjarzadeh A. Antioxidant supplements and semen parameters: An evidence based review. *Int J Reprod Biomed (Yazd).* 2016 Dec;14(12):729-736.

44. Fallah A, Mohammad-Hasani A, Colagar AH. Zinc is an Essential Element for Male Fertility: A Review of Zn Roles in Men's Health, Germination, Sperm Quality, and Fertilization. *J Reprod Infertil.* 2018 Apr-Jun;19(2):69-81.

45. Kothari RP, Chaudhari AR. Zinc Levels in Seminal Fluid in Infertile Males and its Relation with Serum Free Testosterone. *J Clin*

Diagn Res. 2016 May;10(5):CC05-8. doi:
10.7860/JCDR/2016/14393.7723. Epub 2016
May 1.

46. Thakur AS, Littarru GP, Funahashi
I, Painkara US, Dange NS, Chauhan P. Effect
of Ubiquinol Therapy on Sperm Parameters
and Serum Testosterone Levels in
Oligoasthenozoospermic Infertile Men. *J Clin
Diagn Res.* 2015 Sep;9(9):BC01-3. doi:
10.7860/JCDR/2015/13617.6424. Epub 2015
Sep 1.

47. Tiseo BC, Gaskins AJ, Hauser R, Chavarro
JE, Tanrikut C; EARTH Study Team.
Coenzyme Q10 Intake From Food and
Semen Parameters in a Subfertile Population.
Urology. 2017 Apr;102:100-105. doi:
10.1016/j.urology.2016.11.022. Epub 2016
Nov 22.

48. Majzoub A, Agarwal A, Esteves SC.
Antioxidants for elevated sperm DNA
fragmentation: a mini review. *Transl Androl
Urol.* 2017 Sep;6(Suppl 4):S649-S653. doi:
10.21037/tau.2017.07.09.

49. Chavarro JE, Mínguez-Alarcón L, Mendiola
J, Cutillas-Tolín A, López-Espín JJ, Torres-

Cantero AM. Trans fatty acid intake is inversely related to total sperm count in young healthy men. *Hum Reprod.* 2014 Mar;29(3):429-40. doi: 10.1093/humrep/det464. Epub 2014 Jan 12.

50. Çekici H, Akdevelioğlu Y. The association between trans fatty acids, infertility and fetal life: a review. *Hum Fertil (Camb).* 2018 Jan 31:1-10. doi: 10.1080/14647273.2018.1432078.

51. Blasbalg TL, Hibbeln JR, Ramsden CE, Majchrzak SF, Rawlings RR. Changes in consumption of omega-3 and omega-6 fatty acids in the United States during the 20th century. *Am J Clin Nutr.* 2011 May;93(5):950-62. doi: 10.3945/ajcn.110.006643. Epub 2011 Mar 2.

52. Vannice G, Rasmussen H. Position of the academy of nutrition and dietetics: dietary fatty acids for healthy adults. *J Acad Nutr Diet.* 2014 Jan;114(1):136-53. doi: 10.1016/j.jand.2013.11.001.

53. Attaman JA, Toth TL, Furtado J, Campos H, Hauser R, Chavarro JE. Dietary fat and semen quality among men attending a fertility clinic. *Hum Reprod.* 2012

May;27(5):1466-74. doi:
10.1093/humrep/des065. Epub 2012 Mar 13.

54. MInguez-Alarcón L, Chavarro JE, Mendiola
J, Roca M, Tanrikut C, Vioque J, Jørgensen
N, Torres-Cantero AM. Fatty acid intake in
relation to reproductive hormones and
testicular volume among young healthy men.
Asian J Androl. 2017 Mar-Apr;19(2):184-190.
doi: 10.4103/1008-682X.190323.

55. Hosseini B, Nourmohamadi M, Hajipour
S, Taghizadeh M, Asemi Z, Keshavarz
SA, Jafarnejad S. The Effect of Omega-3
Fatty Acids, EPA, and/or DHA
on Male Infertility: A Systematic Review and
Meta-analysis. *J Diet Suppl.* 2018 Feb 16:1-12.

56. National Institute of Health. Omega-3 fatty
acids. Updated June 8, 2018.
https://ods.od.nih.gov/factsheets/Omega3Fa
ttyAcids-Consumer/ Accessed October 16,
2018.

57. Gaskins AJ, Sundaram R, Buck Louis
GM, Chavarro JE. Seafood Intake, Sexual
Activity, and Time to Pregnancy. *J Clin
Endocrinol Metab.* 2018 Jul 1;103(7):2680-2688.
doi: 10.1210/jc.2018-00385.

58. Mínguez-Alarcón L, Afeiche MC, Williams PL, Arvizu M, Tanrikut C, Amarasiriwardena CJ, Ford JB, Hauser R, Chavarro JE; Earth Study Team. Hair mercury (Hg) levels, fish consumption and semen parameters among men attending a fertility center. *Int J Hyg Environ Health*. 2018 Mar;221(2):174-182. doi: 10.1016/j.ijheh.2017.10.014. Epub 2017 Oct 28.

59. Salas-Huetos A, Moraleda R, Giardina S, Anton E, Blanco J, Salas-Salvadó J, Bulló M. Effect of nut consumption on semen quality and functionality in healthy men consuming a Western-style diet: a randomized controlled trial. *Am J Clin Nutr*. 2018 Nov 1;108(5):953-962. doi: 10.1093/ajcn/nqy181.

60. Robbins WA, Xun L, FitzGerald LZ, Esguerra S, Henning SM, Carpenter CL. Walnuts improve semen quality in men consuming a Western-style diet: randomized control dietary intervention trial. *Biol Reprod*. 2012 Oct 25;87(4):101. doi: 10.1095/biolreprod.112.101634. Print 2012 Oct.

61. National Institute of Health. Vitamin D. Updated September 18, 2018. https://ods.od.nih.gov/factsheets/VitaminD-HealthProfessional/. Accessed October 16, 2018.

62. Forrest KY, Stuhldreher WL. Prevalence and correlates of vitamin D deficiency in US adults. *Nutr Res.* 2011 Jan;31(1):48-54. doi: 10.1016/j.nutres.2010.12.001.

63. Rehman R, Lalani S, Baig M, Nizami I, Rana Z, Gazzaz ZJ. Association Between Vitamin D, Reproductive Hormones and Sperm Parameters in Infertile Male Subjects. *Front Endocrinol (Lausanne).* 2018 Oct 16;9:607.

64. de Angelis C, Galdiero M, Pivonello C, Garifalos F, Menafra D, Cariati F, Salzano C, Galdiero G, Piscopo M, Vece A, Colao A, Pivonello R. The role of vitamin D in male fertility: A focus on the testis. *Rev Endocr Metab Disord.* 2017 Sep;18(3):285-305. doi: 10.1007/s11154-017-9425-0.

65. Neville G, Martyn F, Kilbane M, O'Riordan M, Wingfield M, McKenna M, McAuliffe FM. Vitamin D status and fertility outcomes during winter among couples undergoing in

vitro fertilization/intracytoplasmic sperm injection. *Int J Gynaecol Obstet.* 2016 Nov;135(2):172-176. doi: 10.1016/j.ijgo.2016.04.018. Epub 2016 Jul 30.

66. Gaskins AJ, Chavarro JE. Diet and fertility: a review. *Am J Obstet Gynecol.* 2018 Apr;218(4):379-389. doi: 10.1016/j.ajog.2017.08.010. Epub 2017 Aug 24.

67. Academy of Nutrition and Dietetics. What is Vitamin D? Published June 15, 2015.

    https://www.eatright.org/food/vitamins-and-supplements/types-of-vitamins-and-nutrients/what-is-vitamin-d. Accessed November 22, 2018

68. Obeid R, Kirsch SH, Dilmann S, Klein C, Eckert R, Geisel J, Herrmann W. Folic acid causes higher prevalence of detectable unmetabolized folic acid in serum than B-complex: a randomized trial. *Eur J Nutr.* 2016 Apr;55(3):1021-8. doi: 10.1007/s00394-015-0916-z. Epub 2015 May 6.

69. Cole BF, Baron JA, Sandler RS, Haile RW, Ahnen DJ, Bresalier RS, *et al.* Polyp Prevention Study Group. Folic acid for the prevention of colorectal adenomas: a

randomized clinical trial. *JAMA*. 2007 Jun 6;297(21):2351-9.

70. Figueiredo JC, Grau MV, Haile RW, Sandler RS, Summers RW, Bresalier RS, Burke CA, McKeown-Eyssen GE, Baron JA. Folic acid and risk of prostate cancer: results from a randomized clinical trial. *J Natl Cancer Inst*. 2009 Mar 18;101(6):432-5. doi: 10.1093/jnci/djp019. Epub 2009 Mar 10.

71. Morris MS, Jacques PF, Rosenberg IH, Selhub J. Folate and vitamin B-12 status in relation to anemia, macrocytosis, and cognitive impairment in older Americans in the age of folic acid fortification. *Am J Clin Nutr*. 2007 Jan;85(1):193-200.

72. Afeiche MC, Bridges ND, Williams PL, Gaskins AJ, Tanrikut C, Petrozza JC, Hauser R, Chavarro JE. Dairy intake and semen quality among men attending a fertility clinic. *Fertil Steril*. 2014 May;101(5):1280-7. doi: 10.1016/j.fertnstert.2014.02.003. Epub 2014 Mar 14.

73. Chavarro J, Toth T, Sadio S, Hauser R. Soy food and isoflavone intake in relation to semen quality parameters among men from an

infertility clinic. *Hum Reprod.* 2008 Nov; 23(11): 2584–2590.

74. Mínguez-Alarcón L, Afeiche MC, Chiu YH, Vanegas JC, Williams PL, Tanrikut C, Toth TL, Hauser R, Chavarro JE. Male soy food intake was not associated with in vitro fertilization outcomes among couples attending a fertility center. *Andrology.* 2015 Jul;3(4):702-8. doi: 10.1111/andr.12046. Epub 2015 Jun 20.

75. D'Adamo CR, Sahin A. Soy foods and supplementation: a review of commonly perceived health benefits and risks. *Altern Ther Health Med.* 2014 Winter;20 Suppl 1:39-51.

76. Ricci E, Noli S, Ferrari S, La Vecchia I, Cipriani S, De Cosmi V, Somigliana E, Parazzini F. Alcohol intake and semen variables: cross-sectional analysis of a prospective cohort study of men referring to an Italian Fertility Clinic. *Andrology.* 2018 Sep;6(5):690-696. doi: 10.1111/andr.12521. Epub 2018 Jul 18.

77. Li Y, Lin H, Li Y, Cao J. Association between socio-psycho-behavioral factors and male semen quality: systematic review and meta-analyses. *Fertil Steril. 2011;* 95(1);116-123

78. Muthusami KR, Chinnaswamy P. Effect of chronic alcoholism on male fertility hormones

and semen quality. *Fertil Steril.* 2005 Oct;84(4):919-24.

79. Borges E Jr, Braga DPAF, Provenza RR, Figueira RCS, Iaconelli A Jr, Setti AS. Paternal lifestyle factors in relation to semen quality and in vitro reproductive outcomes. *Andrologia.* 2018 Nov;50(9):e13090. doi: 10.1111/and.13090. Epub 2018 Jul 17.

80. Ricci E, Viganò P, Cipriani S, Somigliana E, Chiaffarino F, Bulfoni A, Parazzini F. Coffee and caffeine intake and male infertility: a systematic review. *Nutr J.* 2017;16(1):37. doi: 10.1186/s12937-017-0257-2.

81. Karmon AE, Toth TL, Chiu YH, Gaskins AJ, Tanrikut C, Wright DL, Hauser R, Chavarro JE; Earth Study Team. Male caffeine and alcohol intake in relation to semen parameters and in vitro fertilization outcomes among fertility patients. *Andrology.* 2017 Mar;5(2):354-361. doi: 10.1111/andr.12310. Epub 2017 Feb 10.

82. Ricci E, Noli S, Cipriani S, La Vecchia I, Chiaffarino F, Ferrari S, Mauri PA, Reschini M, Fedele L, Parazzini F. Maternal and Paternal Caffeine Intake and ART Outcomes in Couples Referring to an Italian Fertility

Clinic: A Prospective Cohort. *Nutrients*. 2018 Aug 17;10(8). pii: E1116. doi: 10.3390/nu10081116.

83. Pingitore A, Lima GP, Mastorci F, Quinones A, Iervasi G, Vassalle C. Exercise and oxidative stress: potential effects of antioxidant dietary strategies in sports. *Nutrition*. 2015 Jul-Aug;31(7-8):916-22. doi: 10.1016/j.nut.2015.02.005. Epub 2015 Feb 19.

84. Haijzadeh B, Taribian B, Chehrazi M. The effects of three different exercise modalities on markers of male reproduction in healthy subjects: a randomized controlled trial. *Reproduction*. 2017 Feb;153(2):157-174.

85. Hajizadeh Maleki B, Tartibian B. Resistance exercise modulates male factor infertility through anti-inflammatory and antioxidative mechanisms in infertile men: A RCT. *Life Sci*. 2018 Jun 15;203:150-160. doi: 10.1016/j.lfs.2018.04.039. Epub 2018 Apr 23.

86. Jóźków P, Rossato M. The Impact of Intense Exercise on Semen Quality. *Am J Mens Health*. 2017 May;11(3):654-662. doi: 10.1177/1557988316669045. Epub 2016 Sep 19.

87. Bujan L., Daudin M., Charlet J. P., Thonneau P., Mieusset R. Increase in scrotal temperature in car drivers. Human Reproduction. 2000 Jun;15(6):1355-7.

88. Jung A., Strauss P., Lindner H. J., Schuppe H. C. Influence of moderate cycling on scrotal temperature. *Int J Androl.* 2008 Aug;31(4):403-7.

89. Gebreegziabher Y., Marcos E., McKinon W., Rogers G. Sperm characteristics of endurance trained cyclists. *Int J Sports Med.* 2004 May;25(4):247-51.

90. Kipandula W., Lampiao F. Semen profiles of young men involved as bicycle taxi cyclists in Mangochi District, Malawi: A case-control study. *Malawi Med J.* 2015 Dec;27(4):151-3.

91. Liu MM, Liu L, Chen L, Yin XJ, Liu H, Zhang YH, Li PL, Wang S, Li XX, Yu CH. Sleep Deprivation and Late Bedtime Impair S perm Health Through Increasing Antisperm AntibodyProduction:
A Prospective Study of 981 Healthy Men. *Med Sci Monit.* 2017 Apr 16;23:1842-1848.

92. DHA LA, Rothman KJ, Wesselink AK, Mikkelsen EM, Sorensen HT, McKinnon CJ, Hatch EE. Male sleep duration and fecundability in a North American preconception cohort study. *Fertil Steril.* 2018 Mar;109(3):453-459. doi: 10.1016/j.fertnstert.2017.11.037.

93. Asare-Anane H, Bannison SB, Ofori EK, Ateko RO, Bawah AT, Amanquah SD, Oppong SY, Gandau BB, Ziem JB. Tobacco smoking is associated with decreased semen quality. *Reprod Health.* 2016 Aug 5;13(1):90. doi: 10.1186/s12978-016-0207-z.

94. Practice Committee of the American Society for Reproductive Medicine. Smoking and infertility: a committee opinion. *Fertil Steril.* 2018:110:611-8.

95. Said TM, Ranga G, Agarwal A. Relationship between semen quality and tobacco chewing in men undergoing infertility evaluation. *Fert Steril.* 2005;84(3):649-53.

96. du Plessis SS, Agarwal A, Syriac A. Marijuana, phytocannabinoids, the endocannabinoid system, and male fertility. *J Assist Reprod Genet.* 2015 Nov;32(11):1575-88. doi: 10.1007/s10815-015-0553-8. Epub 2015 Aug 16.

97. Gundersen T.D., Jorgensen N., Andersson A.M., Bang A.K., Nordkap L., Skakkebaek N.E. Association between use of marijuana and male reproductive hormones and semen quality: a study among 1,215 healthy young men. *Am J Epidemiol.* 2015;182:473–481.

98. Carvalho RK, Souza MR, Santos ML, Guimarães FS, Pobbe RLH, Andersen ML, Mazaro-Costa R. Chronic cannabidiol

exposure promotes functional impairment in sexual behavior and fertility of male mice. *Reprod Toxicol.* 2018 Oct;81:34-40. doi: 10.1016/j.reprotox.2018.06.013. Epub 2018 Jun 21.

99. Kasman AM, Thoma ME, McLain AC, Eisenberg ML. Association between use of marijuana and time to pregnancy in men and women: findings from the National Survey of Family Growth. *Fertil Steril.* 2018 May;109(5):866-871. doi: 10.1016/j.fertnstert.2018.01.015. Epub 2018 Mar 16.

100. Wise LA, Wesselink AK, Hatch EE, Rothman KJ, Mikkelsen EM,Sorensen HT, Mahalingaiah S. Marijuana use and fecundability in a North American preconception cohort study. *J Epidemiol Community Health.* 2018 Mar;72(3):208-215. doi: 10.1136/jech-2017-209755. Epub 2017 Dec 22.

101. Hsiao P, Clavijo RI. Adverse Effects of Cannabis on Male Reproduction. *Eur Urol Focus.* 2018 Apr;4(3):324-328.

102. Eisenberg ML. Invited Commentary: The Association Between Marijuana Use and Male

Reproductive Health. *Am J Epidemiol.* 2015 Sep 15;182(6):482-4. doi: 10.1093/aje/kwv137. Epub 2015 Aug 16.

103. Mínguez-Alarcón L, Gaskins AJ, Chiu YH, Messerlian C, Williams PL, Ford JB, Souter I, Hauser R, Chavarro JE. Type of underwear worn and markers of testicular function among men attending a fertility center. *Hum Reprod.* 2018 Sep 1;33(9):1749-1756. doi: 10.1093/humrep/dey259.

104. Avendaño C, Mata A, Sanchez Sarmiento CA, Doncel GF. Use of laptop computers connected to internet through Wi-Fi decreases human sperm motility and increases sperm DNA fragmentation. *Fertil Steril.* 2012 Jan;97(1):39-45.e2. doi: 10.1016/j.fertnstert.2011.10.012. Epub 2011 Nov 23.

105. Zhang G, Yan H, Chen Q, Liu K, Ling X, Sun L, *et al.* Effects of cell phone use on semen parameters: Results from the MARHCS cohort study in Chongqing, China. *Environ Int.* 2016 May;91:116-21. doi: 10.1016/j.envint.2016.02.028. Epub 2016 Mar 4.

106. Yildirim ME, Kaynar M, Badem H, Cavis M, Karatas OF, Cimentepe E. What is

harmful for male fertility: cell phone or the wireless Internet? *Kaohsiung J Med Sci.* 2015 Sep;31(9):480-4. doi: 10.1016/j.kjms.2015.06.006. Epub 2015 Jul 26.

107. Adams JA, Galloway TS, Mondal D, Esteves SC, Mathews F. Effect of mobile telephones on sperm quality: a systematic review and meta-analysis. *Environ Int.* 2014 Sep;70:106-12. doi: 10.1016/j.envint.2014.04.015. Epub 2014 Jun 10.

108. Giwercman A, Rylander L, Lundberg Giwercman Y. Influence of endocrine disruptors on human male fertility. *Reprod Biomed Online.* 2007 Dec;15(6):633-42.

109. Den Hond E, Tournaye H, De Sutter P, Ombelet W, Baeyens W, Covaci A, Cox B, Nawrot TS, Van Larebeke N, D'Hooghe T. Human exposure to endocrine disrupting chemicals and fertility: A case-control study in male subfertility patients. *Environ Int.* 2015 Nov;84:154-60. doi: 10.1016/j.envint.2015.07.017. Epub 2015 Aug 24.

110. Gollenberg AL, Liu F, Brazil C, Drobnis EZ, Guzick D, Overstreet JW, Redmon JB, Sparks A, Wang C, Swan SH. Semen quality in fertile men in relation to psychosocial stress. *Fertil Steril.* 2010 Mar 1;93(4):1104-11. doi: 10.1016/j.fertnstert.2008.12.018. Epub 2009 Feb 24.

111. Ilacqua A, Izzo G, Emerenziani GP, Baldari C, Aversa A. Lifestyle and fertility: the influence of stress and quality of life on male fertility. *Reprod Biol Endocrinol.* 2018 Nov 26;16(1):115. doi: 10.1186/s12958-018-0436-9.

ABOUT THE AUTHOR

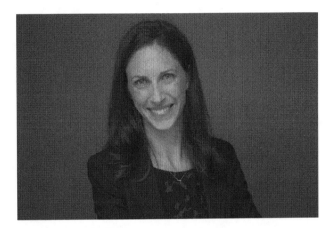

Lauren Manaker is a Registered Dietitian-Nutritionist. She is the founder of Nutrition Now, a virtual private practice in which she provides evidence-based and personalized guidance to people trying to conceive.

Lauren graduated from the University of Florida (Gainesville, FL), where she earned a Bachelor of Science in Food Science and Human Nutrition. She later earned a Master of Science in Clinical Nutrition, and also completed the clinical training program for the Commission on Dietetic Registration at Rush University Medical Center

(Chicago, IL). During her training, she worked as a research assistant at the Center for Disease Control and Prevention (Atlanta, GA), and Shands Hospital (Gainesville, FL).

She later earned a Lactation Educator-Counselor certification from the University of California (San Diego, CA), and a certificate of training on Food Allergies through the Academy of Nutrition and Dietetics.

She has been a member of the Academy of Nutrition and Dietetics (AND) since 2002 and has held leadership positions within the Medical Nutrition Practice Group and Women's Health Practice Group of AND. Lauren's work has been published in peer-reviewed journals and in academy newsletters and books. She has been a reviewer for two AND position papers and has authored many educational book chapters. In 2018, she was the recipient of the prestigious *Emerging Professional in Women's Health Award* from the Women's Health Dietetic Practice Group of the Academy of Nutrition and Dietetics. Lauren currently lives and works in Charleston, SC with her husband Matt, daughter Hannah, and fur-baby Bella.